M000119833

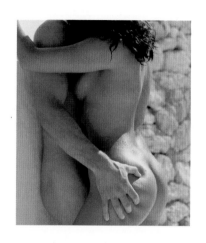

POCKET
KAMA SUTRA
tracey cox

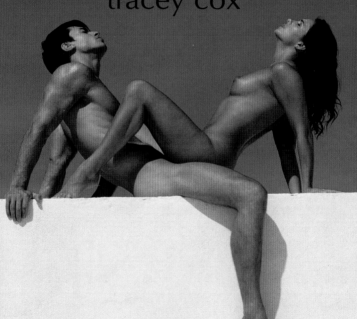

POCKET
KAMA SUTRA
tracey cox

photography by john davis

London, New York, Melbourne, Munich, and Delhi

Editor: Becky Alexander
Design: XAB Design
Project Editor: Daniel Mills
Project Art Editor: Natasha Montgomery
Senior Production Editor: Jenny Woodcock
Production Controller: Hema Gohil
Creative Technical Support: Sonia Charbonnier
Executive Managing Editor: Adèle Hayward
Managing Art Editor: Kat Mead
Art Director: Peter Luff
Publisher: Stephanie Jackson

First published in Great Britain in 2008 by Dorling
Kindersley Limited, 80 Strand, London WC2R 0RL
Penguin Group (UK)

A CIP catalogue record for this book is available from
the British Library
ISBN 978 1 4053 4102 8

Printed and bound in Singapore by Star Standard

It is assumed that couples are monogamous and have
been tested for sexually transmitted infections. Always
practise safe and responsible sex, and consult a doctor
if you have a condition that might preclude strenuous
sexual activity. Challenging intercourse positions might
put a strain on your back or other body parts – do not
attempt them if you have injuries or ailments and
consult your doctor for advice beforehand if you are
concerned. The author and publisher do not accept
any responsibility for any injury or ailment caused by
following any of the suggestions contained in this
book. This is the author's personal interpretation of
ancient spiritual texts like the *Kama Sutra* and is not
intended to be an accurate representation of them.

Discover more at www.dk.com

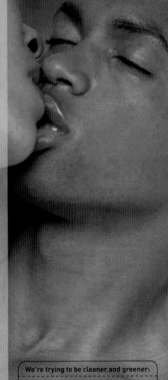

We're trying to be cleaner and greener:

• we recycle waste, switch things off,
give bike loans
• we use paper from responsibly-managed
forests whenever possible
• we ask our printers to actively reduce
water and energy consumption
• we check out our suppliers' working
conditions – they never use child labour

**Find out more about our values and
best practices at www.dk.com**

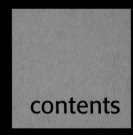

contents

The *Kama Sutra* is a wonderfully quirky, marvellously eccentric, slightly barmy tome, which happens to have **some absolute pearls of sexual wisdom mixed in amongst it all.**

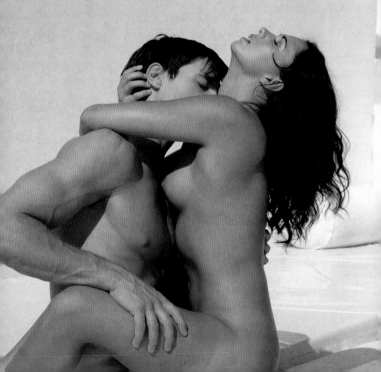

introduction

I put my heart, soul (and other parts I won't mention) into writing this book – but I have to warn you, it's probably nothing like other books you might have read on the *Kama Sutra*. It's irreverent, not terribly spiritual, and I've shamelessly cherry-picked concepts, positions, and techniques from this ancient text. I've reworked, reworded, and quite often taken the mickey out of something some see as spiritually sacred. For this I offer complete and humble apologies. But I did it for a reason.

I've been decidedly sniffy about spiritual sex in the past, but I started researching it for my last book, and was suddenly seized with a need to bring it all to life again and put my own stamp on it. Because I still get the distinct impression most people think of the *Kama Sutra* as a book about sexual positions. It's not. It's a wonderfully quirky, marvellously eccentric, slightly barmy tome, which happens to have some absolute pearls of sexual wisdom mixed in amongst it all. Trouble is, if you do stick to the original wording, a lot of it doesn't seem applicable to modern life – which is why people have a tendency to skip the theory and instead ogle the pictures of people doing erotic acrobatics.

I figured if I rewrote the bits people often miss out on in a way most of us could relate to, you'd be far more likely to actually read them. And if I didn't pretend you had to take it all terribly seriously – because some of it is soooooooo out there, it's impossible not to laugh out loud – you might be even more intrigued. Then I added all the positions you clearly love on top of that, so you didn't feel cheated. And came up with something, I hope, that offers a fresh, innovative twist on the original.

Tracey x

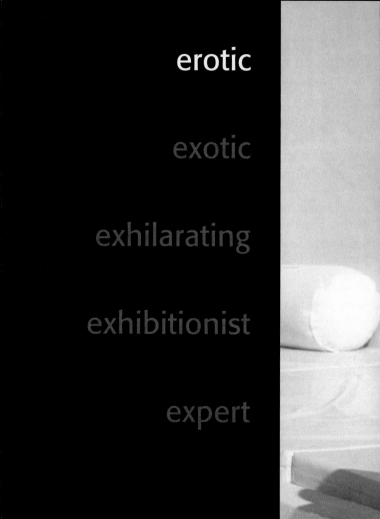

erotic

exotic

exhilarating

exhibitionist

expert

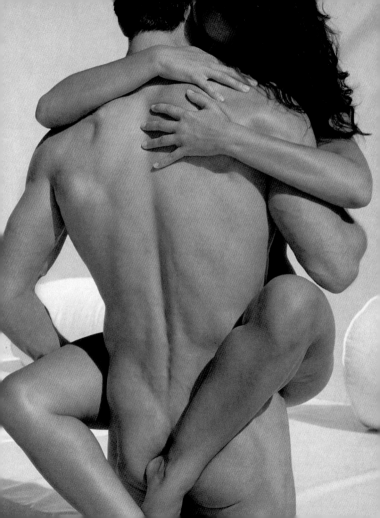

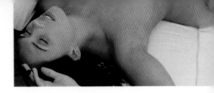

Kama Sutra for dummies

We have all heard of the infamous book the *Kama Sutra*, but how many of us have the foggiest idea of what it's really about? Here's a crash course in the basics of spiritual sex.

Like all things which keep us deliciously intrigued, no one can quite agree on the facts surrounding the original *Kama Sutra*. We know that it was compiled between the first and fourth centuries AD by an elderly Indian sage called Mallanaga Vatsyayana, but little is known of him. Some historians swear he was celibate; others say he got tempted after studying the ancient texts, and went for it!

It's also thought Vatsyayana didn't actually write the *Kama Sutra*, even though he's generally referred to as the author. Folklore says he studied writings of holy men before him and discovered that Nandi, the white bull, stood guard for the mighty gods Shiva and Parvati outside their bedroom while they made love for 10,000 years. (And you thought that 48-hour romp was something worth boasting about!) Nandi swore never to speak of the sex secrets he saw and heard but, just like a fallible human, broke his vow and blabbed. The words he spoke "fell as flowers" and the flowers were gathered, strung onto thread, then woven into a book of 1,000 chapters. As time passed, the book got shortened and eventually condensed to 150 chapters. Vatsyayana managed to compact it into seven parts (only one of which deals exclusively with sex).

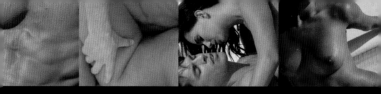

The *Kama Sutra* is basically a guide to life and love. It's addressed to men, but Vatsyayana heartily recommends young women also take a flick through before marriage (with their fiancé's consent, of course!). At the time the *Kama Sutra* was written, there was no shame associated with sex – Hindus thought sex wasn't just natural and necessary, but sacred. A veritable shagfest apparently! (Time machine, anyone?)

In 1883, the *Kama Sutra* was translated by two English adventurers: Sir Richard Burton and Forster Fitzgerald Arbuthnot. So risqué was it for the Western world, they had to create their own company to publish it. Even then, it was only available through subscription and mainly read by scholars or upper class "gents" with an appetite for erotica. Published on general release in the US and UK in 1962, it has remained the world's most famous sex book, even if most people are under the misconception that it's a "positions book" with lots of naughty drawings.

At the time the *Kama Sutra* was written, there was **no shame associated with sex**. Hindus thought sex wasn't just natural and necessary, but sacred. **A veritable shagfest apparently!**

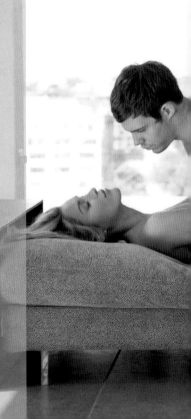

01

TOP KAMA SUTRA POSITION

rising

Spreading her thighs ups the eroticism, and being able to make eye contact adds intimacy to passion.

How to do it

She raises her legs in the air, making a wide "V" shape by holding her thighs open with her hands. He penetrates in the usual man-on-top position. Penetration is already pretty intense, but if she's feeling particularly raunchy and wants him even deeper, she should bend her knees and bring them up to her chest. Some interpretations of this pose include her putting her feet in front of him and pressing them against the top of his chest.

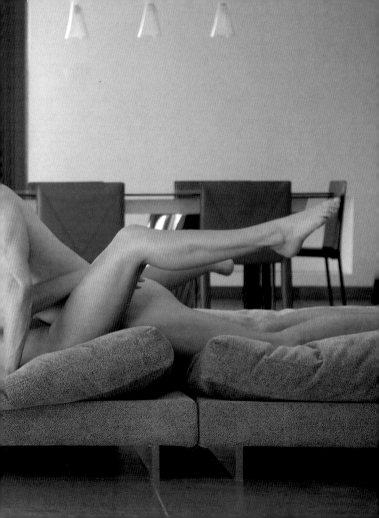

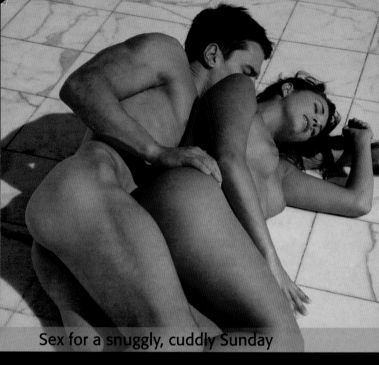

Sex for a snuggly, cuddly Sunday

SLEEPY SPOONS

Perfect for half-asleep-hungover Sunday morning sex, or post-boozy Sunday lunch sessions! This position is remarkably intimate, even though you're both facing in the same direction, because there's full body contact. He penetrates from behind, and she lifts her bottom and/or uses her hands to help him. He can kiss or bite her neck, easily reaching around to play with her breasts or clitoris. It's a great position if you're pregnant!

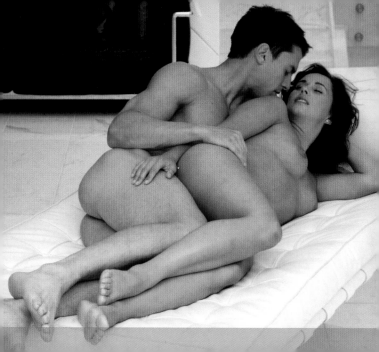

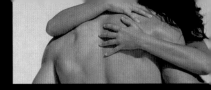

debonking the myth

Does tantra deserve the hype? Is the *Kama Sutra* a sacred sex manual or an out-dated old textbook? Before we get any further into specifics, I thought a broad overview of what I think works and what doesn't, might be useful. That way we'll both know where we're coming from – and can get on to the business of coming.

As I've already mentioned, I was a late convert to spiritual sex. Being a rather impatient person (okay, drop the "rather"), reports of tediously long intercourse sessions had little appeal. Gazing into a lover's eyes for a minute or two might be sweet but, quite frankly, I'd be mentally tossing up which film to watch after that. As for things like inhaling my partner's breath… well, that still makes a little bit of sick rise in my throat.

Being a huge fan of gloriously animal, throw-each-other-around-a-bit sex, the controlled element of spiritual sex also put me off. But – and it's a big

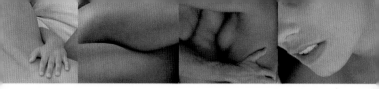

WHAT WORKS

It promotes foreplay A basic rule of spiritual sex is to insist he waits until she is trembling with desire before even thinking about intercourse. There are also lots of erotic kissing techniques, and Vatsyayana also recognized female orgasm ahead of his time.

It isn't orgasm focused While orgasm is recognized as a type of nirvana, *Kama Sutra* sex is unhurried, with no pressure or official "finish". All the spiritual texts have a healthy disregard for the standard pattern of modern sex – a bit of kissing then the missionary position. Let's be honest: anything else is an improvement.

It keeps sex exciting If there's one resounding message from spiritual sex, it's that couples need to put lots of effort into their sex lives. Put a tenth of the effort into your sex life suggested by the *Kama Sutra*, and it'll be one hundred times more effort than the average couple.

There's more than one way to thrust He's encouraged to try lots of thrusting techniques, choosing whatever suits the mood.

WHAT DOESN'T WORK

Ejaculation is discouraged It's true that orgasm and ejaculation are separate processes, but the spiritualists take it further and say the loss of semen weakens a man. Not true. Silly.

Sexual rituals If you're the sort who likes a bit of pomp and ceremony, this may appeal. Others will want to skip the pre-sex rituals for a quickie.

Lengthy sex sessions It's not a myth that spiritual sex can go on for one or two hours. This is for meditation and an exchange of vital energies. Yes, it forces you to stay in the moment, but you might get bored silly.

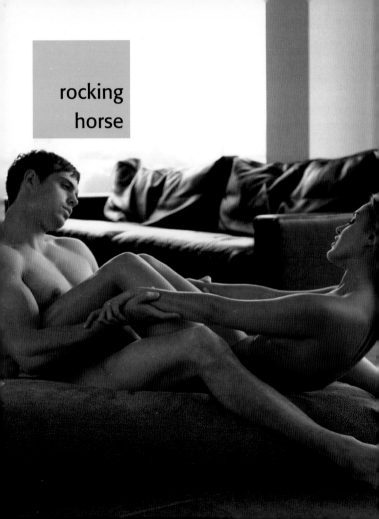

rocking
horse

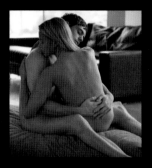

<<STEP ONE

He sits with legs stretched out, she sits sideways between his legs, with her legs over his thigh. Both hug and enjoy the flesh-to-flesh contact. Enjoy the intimacy.

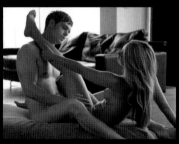

<<STEP FOUR

Clasp each other's wrists, then both lean backward. Move into a rocking horse motion, pulling each other up with your arms.

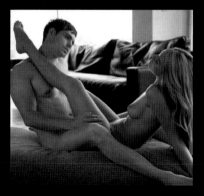

^STEP TWO

She provocatively places her ankle on his shoulder and holds her calf muscle. Show off that flexibility girl!

<<STEP THREE

He's – hurrah! – allowed to penetrate. She leans back supporting her own weight, and lifts her bottom. No thrusting yet though!

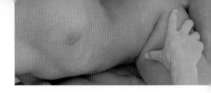

sex like it used to be

The *Kama Sutra* says foreplay begins way before the first touch or kiss. The ancient Hindus were as body-conscious as they were hedonistic – Vatsyayana gives explicit and lengthy instructions on personal hygiene. A man should "bathe daily, anoint his body with oil every other day, get his head shaved every four days, and the sweat of the armpits should also be removed." (Very good idea, that last suggestion.) Once both partners were suitably bathed and shaved, they would meet in the "pleasure room". This sumptuous sex pit was decorated with flowers, fragrant with perfume – and came with a fully stocked bar and hors d'oeuvres. Excellent! While eating and drinking "freely" (getting sloshed), the couple would carry on "amusing conversations" on various subjects (chat each other up) and might "also talk suggestively of things which would be considered as coarse" (talk dirty).

Basically, Vatsyayana is describing a sex session which has been planned, anticipated, and enjoyed. The sort of sex you had at the beginning of your relationship. Fact: people fall out of lust when sex is taken for granted. And they fall out of love if they're not having good, regular sex. If you want sex to be as good as it was at the start (and who doesn't?) give it and each other the same amount of attention you did then. It wasn't just hormones and the feel of fresh flesh, the sex was good because you gave it priority. Take a page out of the *Kama Sutra* and aim for at least one "special" sex session a month.

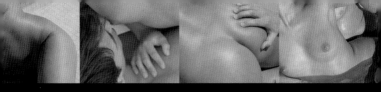

THINGS TO TRY

Make your bedroom sexy Keep it at the right temperature with low, flattering lighting (tea-lights on plates on the floor work well). Burn oils or scented candles, put some music on. The Kama Sutra encourages you to involve all five senses in sex – not just touch and sight.

Make yourselves sexy Get yourselves out of those trackpants and slide into something less comfortable – and sexier!

Have some "treat" nibbles in bed Eat these and have a glass of bubbly either before or after sex.

Brush or play with each other's hair Rather handily, you can do this one while watching TV.

Take a page out of the *Kama Sutra* and aim for at least **one "special" sex session a month.**

Have a bath together Soap each other's bodies and dry each other off afterward. Wash each other's hair. Lots of people find this sexy, particularly if it involves a nice head massage.

Give each other a massage Massages, like kissing, tend to happen at the start of a relationship, then peter out rapidly. Resurrect them. The Kama Sutra shows pictures of men pleasuring their partner's clitoris using their big toe. Why not give this a go as well? And then why not do it under the tablecloth next time you're at a posh restaurant?

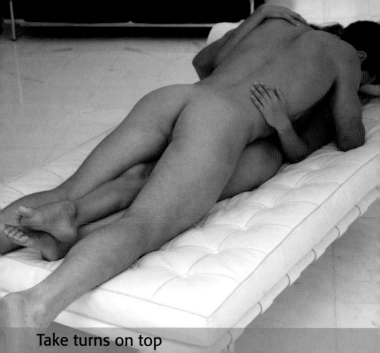

Take turns on top

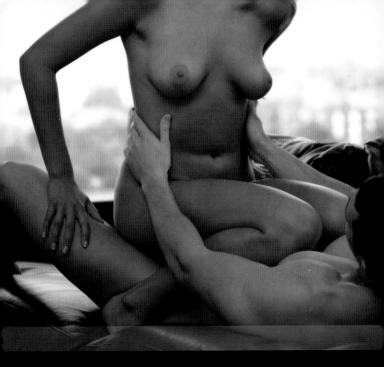

THE BEE

Feeling particularly strong? Try the bee. It looks easy, but you need strength and practice to master it. He lies on his back and she jumps on top, feet flat on the bed beside his hips then, holding his knees for support and leverage, swings her hips both left and right over his penis, hovering in sensual circles, just as a bee floats above a flower. It's all about varying her hip movements to produce exquisite sensations for both of you.

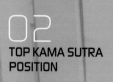

pressed

She lies back in a sexily submissive pose, giving him a fabulous bird's-eye view of the action.

How to do it

Put both feet against his chest, and hang on to the top of his thighs to keep your groins pulled close. He holds on to her feet to hold her steady. This position shortens and tightens the vagina, for a snug fit.

It's also perfect for practising your thrusting techniques. Try a mix of deep and shallow thrusts for starters. He also gets a prime view of his penis sliding in and out of her as he's performing.

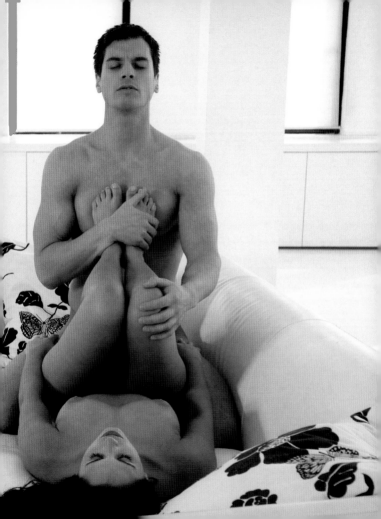

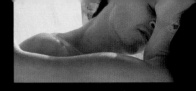

kick-ass kissing

The *Kama Sutra* turns kissing into an art form. It doesn't just tell you how to kiss (in painstaking detail), it tells you where, when, and what type of kiss to use. Kissing is seen as a powerful tool to manipulate your lover and get your needs met. There is a kiss if you want to wake your partner for morning sex ("the kiss that kindles love" involves planting one on them while they're sleeping to show you're in the mood for sex) and a kiss when you're feeling needy and they're not paying you enough attention ("the kiss that turns away").

The *Kama Sutra* turns **kissing into an art form.** It doesn't just tell you **how to kiss** (in painstaking detail), it tells you **where, when, and what type of kiss to use.**

Fancy a bit? A woman who places her head on a man's thigh while bathing him, then gives a little kiss on the thigh, has landed "a demonstrative kiss" designed to "inflame" him.

There are lots of fancy names for standard smackers as well. The "throbbing" kiss, for instance, is simply a kiss where you move the lower lip but not the top one. The "bent" kiss sounds magnificently kinky, but in fact means your faces are at an angle to each other. "Tongue fighting" is simply our version of French kissing.

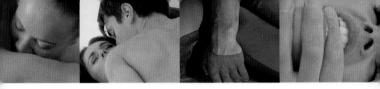

CLEVER KISSING TECHNIQUES WORTH TRYING

Considering the tongue contains more nerves and muscles than almost any other part of the body, it's not hard to figure out why tongue-tussling features strongly in our sexuality today.

The eye lock Make loads of eye contact during kissing and you add both intimacy and eroticism to the whole thing.

Get licking Explore their whole face – lick their eyelids, ears, and underside of the chin. Sounds yucky? Give it a go.

Get sucking Suck their tongue, lick the inside of their lips, nip their lips with your teeth. Suck each other's tongues simultaneously – hard – when you're both on the verge of orgasm. Insert your fingers as you lick and suck on their mouth, and let them suck on them as well.

Keep kissing erotically after either of you orgasm and you're much more likely to keep going and enjoy seconds.

Thrust with your tongue Do this to imitate intercourse, while you're having intercourse to make sure they're really concentrating.

Pull back Pause between kisses to read their expression and make eye contact. When they lunge back in, hold back for a few seconds to tease.

Make a kiss soulful or raunchy Cradle their face in your hands to keep it romantic. To make it passionate, hold their arms above their head with one hand and explore their body with your other hand while you kiss.

Soul kissing This is incredibly intimate so best save it for a long-term lover! Get your partner to masturbate to orgasm while you kiss them intensely and erotically. Then, before climax, pull back, hold their face in your hands, and look deep into their eyes.

erotic

exotic

exhilarating

exhibitionist

expert

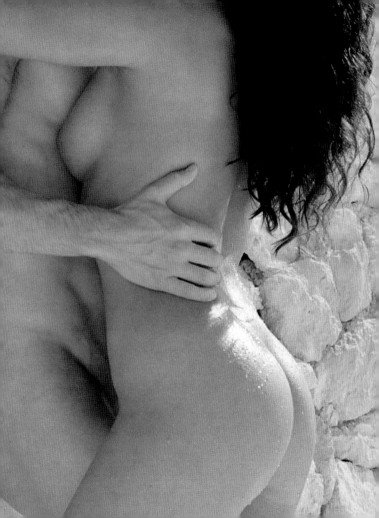

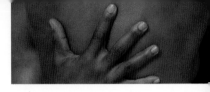

exotic, erotic embraces

There is loads of detail in the *Kama Sutra* even for such simple things as a cuddle. Vatsyayana saw life as something to be understood and mastered, which ultimately meant taking everything apart and examining all the elements to figure out how it all worked. To him, a hug isn't just a hug, it sends a myriad of signals to both participants. After analyzing celebrity couples' body language for years – based heavily on hugs (or the lack of them) – I have to say, I heartily agree. A cuddle is never just a cuddle – there is a message in each and every one of them. Tentative and charged: By God I fancy you. Warm and close: I love you. Stiff and distant: I'm angry with you. Has our snuggling and cuddling style changed over the past, ohh 2,000 years? Surprisingly, less than you think: there are lessons to be learnt. I've put six embraces to the test:

A cuddle is never just a cuddle – there is a message in each and every one of them.

1. The touching embrace
Kama Sutra: He "accidentally" brushes up against her and touches her on the front or the side.
Today: Lust-struck lovers often deliberately put their hands, thighs, or feet close to a longed-for person and pretend a touch was accidental. You can definitely try this one at home.

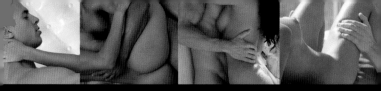

2. The piercing embrace
Kama Sutra: She bends over, as if to pick something up from the ground, her breasts touch him, and he fondles them.
Today: Best tone this one down a tad. Fondling breasts before actually asking someone out isn't done (except in fantasy). Caress with eyes only.

3. The rubbing embrace
Kama Sutra: You're out strolling in public and your bodies rub up against each other.
Today: Nothing new there then.

4. The pressing embrace
Kama Sutra: Overcome by lust, one of you pushes the other up against a wall or pillar.
Today: Pillars might be in short supply, but fridges work just as well.

5. Twining like a creeper
Kama Sutra: Standing, she clings closely, like a vine to a tree, pulls his face down to hers, and looks lovingly at him, desperate to be kissed.
Today: He'll be snogging your face off in a matter of seconds.

6. Mixing sesame seeds with rice
Kama Sutra: Lying down hugging closely in a tangle of arms and legs, rubbing thighs together.

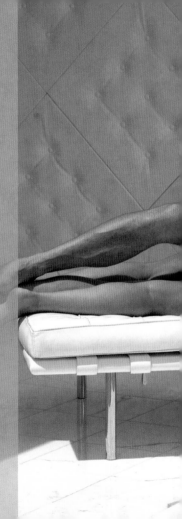

side-by-side

Face-to-face, intense eye contact, snuggled in each other's arms… this is more like an erotic cuddle than full-blown sex.

How to do it

A fantastic position to introduce a reluctant lover to spiritual sex. Start in the good old missionary position – him on top – then once he's penetrated, roll onto your sides, wrapping your arms around each other for support, his thigh straddling her hip. Don't attempt conventional thrusting here, instead squeeze those pelvic floor muscles and enjoy more subtle thrusting movements, and the intimacy.

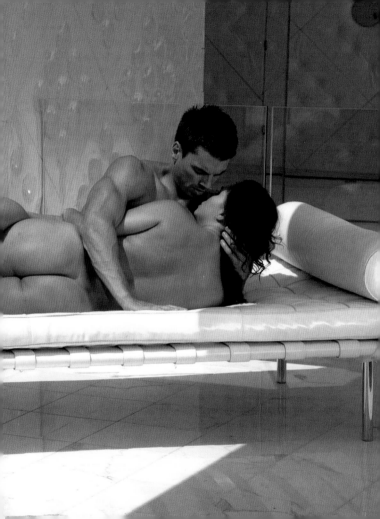

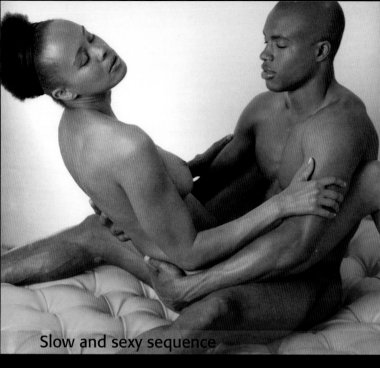

Slow and sexy sequence

LOVERS' LINK

He sits with legs extended and apart. She lowers herself on top,
allowing him to penetrate, before sitting on his lap. She clasps
his upper arms, he supports her back. This pose isn't actually
intended to provide an orgasm for each of you, rather a relaxing
way to simply enjoy being sexually linked. Again, it's all about
appreciating each sexual feeling for its own worth rather than
thinking all roads lead to intercourse.

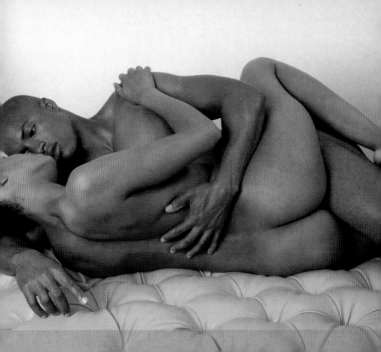

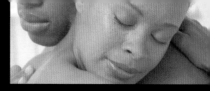

sex with soul

Modern society tends to separate sex and love – spiritual sex works on reuniting the two. If you'd like sex which merges raunch and romance, you've come to the right place!

There's a moment during orgasm when the rest of the world around you ceases to exist. For those precious few seconds, you are 100 per cent truly, utterly, and exclusively concentrated on what you are experiencing. Simultaneously immersed, drowning, floating in pleasure. Now just imagine if you could make that feeling last almost the entire time you are having sex – and your partner is in that bubble with you. That's soul sex.

Want some? Thought you might. Thing is, while we like to pretend we're fascinated purely by the exotic positions in the *Kama Sutra*, it's also because it hints at a different type of sex – sex which is a hell of a lot better than what we're currently having. Spiritual sex requires a

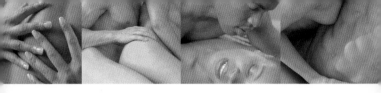

MAKE EVERYDAY SEX SPIRITUAL

These are small but significant ways you can turn wham-bam-thank-you-ma'am sex into something with a little more depth and feeling.

Stop thinking of sex as a physical activity Instead think of it as a way of connecting your minds and souls as well as your bodies.

Imagine you're exchanging energy Even if you honestly don't believe (as the spiritualists do) that you can move sexual energy around your body at will, you can't argue with the concept of it. It's really just another term to describe arousal and feeling turned on.

Maintain eye contact during sex Most of us close our eyes during sex to concentrate on the sensations of what's happening to our body. Others do it because they feel faintly embarrassed. It does feel a bit weird and over-intimate at the start, but once you get past the initial discomfort it's deeply sexy and you do feel a lot more connected. If you can't maintain contact the whole way through, take baby steps and try it for short bursts of time.

Match your breathing While exchanging breaths – you inhale what they're exhaling and vice versa – doesn't appeal to the squeamish, breathing in time is simple and effective. It's calming, slows you down, and does make you feel more "as one".

Have sex without a goal Stop judging the success of your sessions by how many or how intense your orgasms were or how many positions you tried. Stop thinking of sex as having a beginning (foreplay), a middle (intercourse), and an end (orgasm). Instead, think of it as a time when you're going to pleasure each other and be connected.

clasping

If this looks familiar, that's because it is! It's another name for that old faithful, the missionary position.

How to do it

When you fancy getting up close and personal, you can't beat just climbing on top! Which is basically what's happening here: she lies flat on her back with legs apart, he jumps on top and enters and – *voilà!* – you've just assumed the staple sex position for pretty much every couple worldwide. There's a reason why it's so popular: you can lick, bite, and kiss each other, and whisper wicked things. You can also do it anywhere, any time…

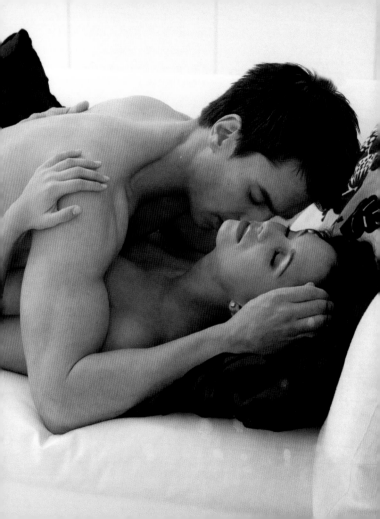

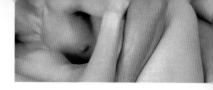

muscle up

Practise all you like, but you aren't going to come close (or at all) if you don't get a firm grip on yourself. Like, literally. Here's all you need to know about the secret strengtheners that really do make all the difference.

You'll both require a reasonable level of physical fitness to master spiritual sex, but I'm actually not just talking limb flexibility or stamina: you need to be skilled at muscle control. We talk a lot about pelvic muscle control for women, but did you know that men can achieve multiple orgasms by delaying or withholding ejaculation via control of their PC (pubococcygeal) muscle? The concept of multiple orgasms for men has never really caught on, probably because it requires holding off. But, if you want a truly brilliant bam-chicka-wow-wow good time that results in your girlfriend looking at you with limpid, liquid eyes, this could provide it.

Your PC muscles form a triangular shape, which stretches from the penis to the anus in men and from the front of the vulva to the anus in women. The benefits of both men and women doing regular PC "pull-ups" are immense. The fitter and more toned this muscle, the greater the sensation for both of you. The vagina grips the penis nice and tightly, making it better for him and intensifying orgasms for her. The exercises also increase arousal because they improve the blood flow to the pelvic area, upping lubrication. So even if you don't achieve the jackpot of multiple orgasms for both of you, regular workouts pay off big time.

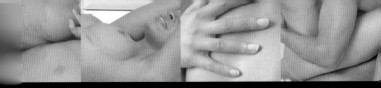

FOR HIM

Here's what you're basically doing in a sentence: squeezing and releasing the same muscle which stops you peeing, makes your bottom squeeze tight, and your penis lift. There! That's not so difficult is it?

1. Inhale and focus on your PC muscle.
2. Exhale and contract the muscle.
3. Inhale and relax.
4. Repeat 10 times, 3 or 4 times a day. (You can't overdo it.)

ADVANCED STUFF

If you feel close to ejaculation, squeeze that PC as strongly as you can and breathe deeply. This should (with practice) delay ejaculation.

FOR HER

When a woman contracts her muscles during intercourse, it's known as "the pair of tongs" in the Kama Sutra. To check if you're doing it correctly and/or improving, put a finger you-know-where and squeeeeze!

1. Breathe in and deliberately relax the area around your vagina and anus.
2. Breathe out and draw up the area until you feel a lifting sensation.
Repeat 10–20 times, 3–4 times a day.

ADVANCED STUFF

During intercourse, squeeze and relax throughout to "milk" the penis. You can also pump your "chi" (vital energy that flows through your body, supplying energy to your organs) for a full body orgasm!

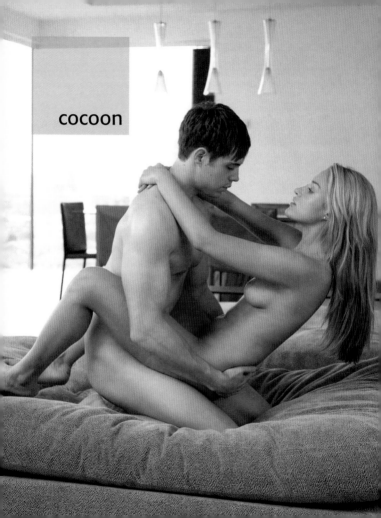

cocoon

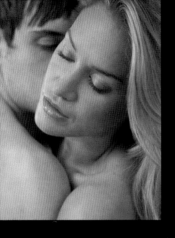

<<STEP ONE

Simply hug, breathing in unison and appreciating each other. It's supposed to be a gentle "let's connect on a spiritual level" one, but you can hot things up by kissing. Stay in the moment, at least for a few minutes.

^V^VSTEP TWO

He kneels, she climbs on top, continuing to cuddle. He's now inside her, but no thrusting just yet! This is all about merging as one, feeling "cocooned".

<<STEP THREE

Now you can get on to some real action… She leans back and he lifts her high off the bed and on to his thighs. She hangs on to his neck for support as he begins moving her back and forth to create some much-longed for friction. Move in close again if you fancy snogging (and who doesn't?)

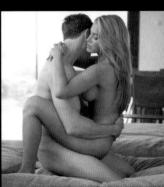

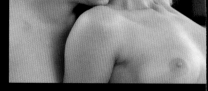

posh new ways to push

A new thrusting style can transform tried-and-tired sex into a fresh, feisty passionate encounter. This is one area where the *Kama Sutra* is particularly inspiring, offering up not one but 10 different thrusting strokes for you to choose from, although I don't suggest you attempt all these techniques in one session – we want you to look sexy, not like Elvis on speed.

If there's one area where most men are lazy with a capital "L", it's with their thrusting technique: in-out-in-out (yawn) in-out. Same speed, same depth, same hip motion, same bloody everything. Because traditional thrusting is so much the norm, it doesn't take a lot to impress us. A slight, sexy swivel combined with a grinding, circular motion and you're elevated to Best Lover Ever, so go on give it some variety.

I don't suggest you attempt all these techniques in one session – **we want you to look sexy, not like Elvis on speed.**

TOP THRUSTING TECHNIQUES
Churning He grasps his penis at the base and moves it in circles inside the vagina. Another variation that scores mega brownie points: he holds his penis and flicks the (oh-so-soft) head of his penis over her clitoris until she's close to orgasm. At the last minute, he penetrates and, still holding his penis, "churns" it in circles.

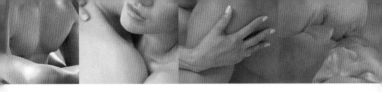

Double-edged sword He strikes sharply downwards into the vagina, away from the G-spot. This is a totally different sensation and, remember, the Kama Sutra isn't orgasm focused so has different aims.

Rubbing She raises her hips by putting a pillow under her bum, and he thrusts in a rising (upward) motion. This makes everything more accessible and alters angles with interesting results.

Pressing The original text says he should press his penis "excitedly" into her womb and hold it there. This is to decrease the level of excitement and delay ejaculation while everyone calms down.

Buffeting He pulls out completely and then penetrates again with a fast, hard stroke. Some women (like me) wince rather than melt at the thought of this. Careful if you aren't overly keen on deep penetration.

Boar's blow He puts continuous pressure on one side of the vagina. Try both – one side may be more sensitive than the other.

Bull's blow He thrusts wildly in all directions like a bull tossing his horns. It should go without saying that attempting this one too early on could mean the whole thing is over before she can say, "That feels grea…". Also not a great one for first-time sex: you might look like a loon.

Sporting of a sparrow He makes rapid, shallow in-and-out strokes. Not good if he is close to climax… oops, see what I mean?

Sparrow's play He quivers inside her vagina, usually just before orgasm. No need to practise this one really, it just happens usually.

Love's tailor He inserts just the head of his penis and makes several small in and out tiny thrusts. Then, suddenly, in a single stroke, he thrusts the whole of the penis into her. The idea is to accomplish several sets of these, but don't be surprised if you lose it at the first fence.

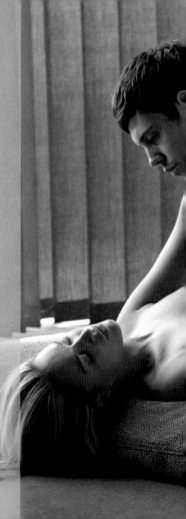

twining

He might be on top, but
winding a leg around his
thigh puts her in command
of the action for a soul-to-
soul sexual smooch.

How to do it

The small, but spiritually significant
variation on the standard face-to-
face position makes a big difference.
She places one leg across his thigh
to draw him as close to her as
possible – and puts herself in the
power position because she can
now use pressure from her heel to
guide the depth, rhythm, and pace
of penetration. Up the difficulty by
doing this position standing up.

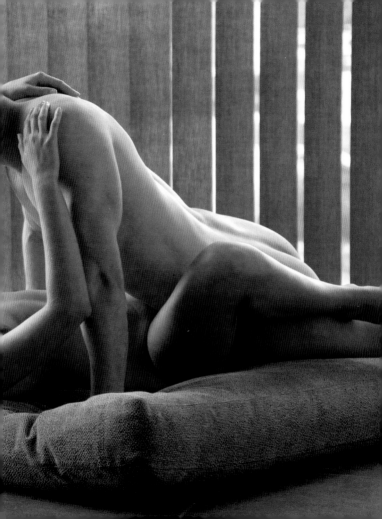

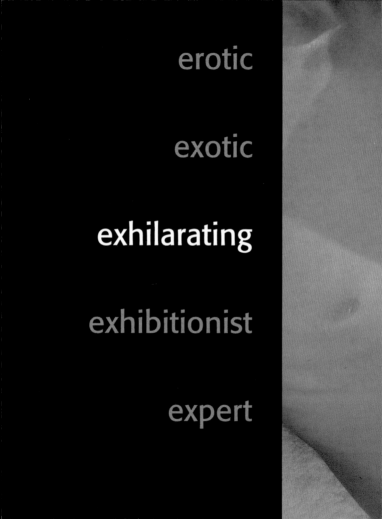

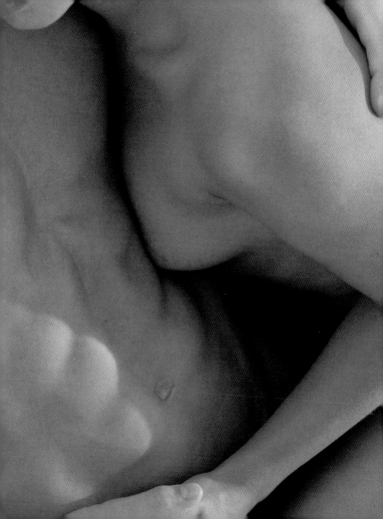

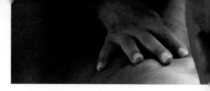

get a grip: hand-jobs for him

His hand and his penis probably already have a very close relationship, which is why they say you can never give a guy a hand-job better than he can give himself. Unless it's the type he couldn't possibly do solo…

The *Kama Sutra* is devoted to the pursuit of pleasure and you're encouraged to treat each sexual act in isolation, not as something that gets you one step closer to intercourse. Using your hand to take him right through to orgasm, rather than as a prelude to other things, is something women tend to do at the start of a relationship – particularly during the "let's wait before having full sex" part. Fear of being thought "easy" might stop us proceeding to the penetration stage, but refusing to lend him a helping hand in the meantime seems impolite. Hence a hand-job is usually the first sexual act a couple experience. Trouble is, once oral sex and intercourse elbow their way into the bedroom, hand-jobs seem to go out of the window. Spiritual sex devotees say bollocks to that! Well, they probably wouldn't say bollocks, but they would throw their hands up in horror at today's waste of a sexual act that can be a star attraction in itself.

However, he'll be losing out if you use the same hand techniques every time. Need a few tricks to freshen up a tired repertoire? Try some of the ones on the next few pages. Every single one works *much* better with lube, by the way. So squeeze some onto your hands, and rub them together to warm it up before working some magic.

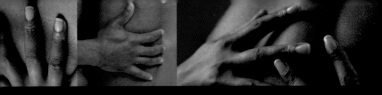

HAD A SNIP?

You'll need to adjust the techniques depending on whether he's circumcised or uncircumcised. If he's "uncut", he'll be a lot more sensitive because the head of his penis is covered by skin and not exposed to things like rubbing against clothing. Start gently if this is the case and ask him for feedback. Get him to show you how he does it himself and imitate his technique. The trick is to put your hand in exactly the same place and position as he does at the very start. Uncut guys tend to put their hands lower on the shaft, cut men often grip nearer the head.

His hand and penis already have a very close relationship, so if you want to beat him at his own game, try some moves he can't do himself.

ENCORE, ENCORE!

Quite early into your sex session, give him an orgasm with your hand, let him concentrate on you for a little while, then use your hand to get him aroused again. He's got more chance of lasting longer during penetration second time around. An effective technique to stop him climaxing too soon: push on his "million dollar point" and get him to squeeze his PC muscle at the same time. You'll find it by inserting a finger inside his bottom, up to the first joint, and searching for a small indentation.

THE HAND-JOB TECHNIQUES

Here are some ideas to add some spice to your usual routine. And if you haven't given him a hand-job for a long time, he is going to love this!

Blow-up doll Weave your hands together and interlock your thumbs leaving a space in the middle, rather like a "fake vagina". With his penis snuggled nicely inside, move your hand up and down keeping a firm grip. Add a twist for extra effect.

Floppy fixer If he's not very erect, take a firm grip at the base of his penis and squeeze while pulling upward, working up the full length. When you reach the head, repeat the same motion using the other hand and continue alternating hands.

Member massage Put your hands on either side of his penis and press it flat against his belly. Now use your thumbs to massage up and down the middle of the shaft.

Wind him up Link your fingers together and put your hands around the base of his penis. Start moving them up the shaft, twisting them continuously from side to side, left to right. Move them around so you're reaching new areas.

The big squeeze Wait until he's got a hard erection then take a firm grip, clasping your hand at the top of the shaft. Position your fingers so they're nudged up against the corona (the ridge separating the head from the shaft) then squeeze. Hold the squeeze for a second, release, then repeat. Combine it with a more conventional movement.

Boy scout Pretend you're a boy scout trying to start a fire by rolling a stick between your hands. Hold the palms of your hands straight, facing either side of his penis and using the rolling/rubbing motion, start at the bottom and slide upward, then down again, keeping a consistent rhythm. Start slowly, then build pressure and speed when he approaches climax.

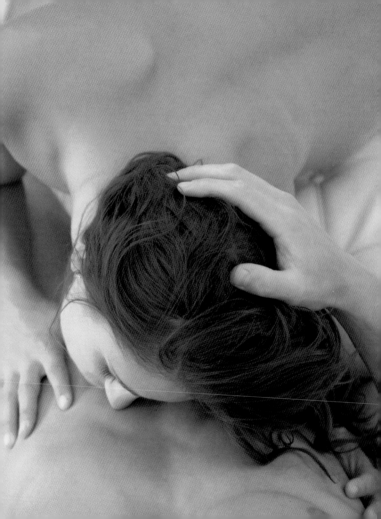

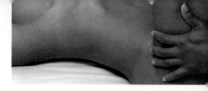

heavenly hand-jobs for her

Rubbing a woman's "yoni" until it becomes "soft" gets a definite thumbs up from the *Kama Sutra*. Most men know how to give your bog-standard hand-job, and I bet your fingers make a bee-line for her clitoris. However, ancient Taoists believed there were three "gates" of pleasure on the female body. And here's exactly what to do with each of them…

THE FIRST GATE – THE CLITORIS
The clitoris gets No. 1 spot. This is the part you already know lots about (if not, why not?), so I'm going to go straight into it…

Ditch lying beside her Sit behind her, get her to sit between your legs and lie back against you, then reach around to find her clitoris. Or bend her over a table or sofa and kiss her neck as you finger her from behind.
How wet is she? Add lubricant if necessary, to make things nice and slippery, then gently part her lips with your fingers and move into the basic stroke: letting your middle finger run back and forth between the inner lips, gently skimming the clitoris each time.
Vary the strokes Switch to sitting in front of her and now hold two fingers in a V-shape around her clitoris, then let your fingers move into a rocking motion. Press them down, using medium pressure, then pull back, then press down – and repeat in a smooth, continuous motion.
As she nears orgasm Get her to bear down (push out with her pelvic muscles) to increase the sensation.

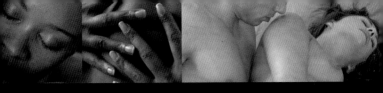

THE SECOND GATE – THE G-SPOT

OK, this time we're going for something new: "internal ejaculation". What the hell is it? It's the ancient Taoist version of the modern world's female ejaculation. Why go there? Well, along with a blissful feeling of "release", her orgasms will be more intense. Which (along with giving her more of them) is the name of the game, right? The benefit to you? Well, she's going to want more of them…

The fluid females ejaculate spiritual-style is rather romantically called "the nectar of the moon". Unlike our culture, which tends to be repulsed rather than delighted by her "lurve" juices, ancient lovers were positively eager to taste and absorb the "yin" (vaginal) essence because of its many benefits. Today it's exactly the opposite – I get lots of letters from women who are mortified rather than thrilled if they're the ones causing the wet patch, convinced their partner will think they've wet themselves!

Here's the challenge, guys: it's your job to make her feel comfortable enough to give this a try because it's going to be a hell of an experience for both of you. The orgasm she'll have really will qualify as spiritual, because it'll be out of this world. In order to let it happen, she must allow herself to lose control – and that's something which lots of women find difficult. So before you move on to the physical stuff, make sure her head's in the right place. You can do this by making her feel loved, secure, sexually adored, and by letting her know you won't ever judge her. Get her to repeat after you: "The only thing that can happen if I let go, is pleasure!"

One final thing: if she doesn't ejaculate, don't feel like you've failed. Ejaculation is a hotly contended issue, with some dismissing it entirely, others embracing it, and others saying only certain women can do it. Rest assured, an orgasm is pretty much guaranteed, even if ejaculation isn't.

Get her to repeat after you: **"The only thing that can happen if I let go, is pleasure!"**

G-spot orgasms However spectacular they are, these involve getting through a not-so-pleasant period where she's absolutely convinced she's about to pee (it's because you're pressing on the urethra). Get her to pee first, so psychologically she knows there's no urine in her bladder.

Get her to sit between your legs Reach around to touch her – or bend her over something and work from behind.

Insert your finger Use lube if she needs it, then make a "pulling" motion (like you're beckoning someone over). Use your middle finger – it's usually the longest – and use the others to work on her clitoris. You're attempting to find a small, spongy area which feels ridgy and becomes more raised the more it's stimulated.

Start massaging the area Use more pressure than you would on the clitoris, and alternate massage with the "come here" finger motion. Rather than working around the area, like you would the clitoris at the start, keep massaging directly on the spot and keep going. (I don't care if the game has started – consistency is the key.)

Encourage her to breathe slowly and deeply As she feels the pressure build, get her to deliberately relax her pelvic floor muscles rather than tensing them.

THE THIRD GATE – THE CERVIX

The AFE (anterior fornix erogenous zone) lies deep inside the vagina – and I mean deep. It's through stimulation of this area – or even the cervix itself – that her third sensational orgasm can be produced. As with the G-spot, you need fingers like ET or a vibrator/dildo to get to it, or you can reach the AFE relatively easily during intercourse. The best positions to try: she lies on her tummy and you lie on top of her; or she jumps on top, leaning back rather than forward. Get this right and the contractions she feels are strong – and addictive. Unlike the clitoris, the area doesn't get over-sensitive after the first climax. Which, of course, means she's going to want more, and more. I'm going to finish up this section by giving you the famous "multi-tasker". It's designed to hit all three gates as well, and add a fourth dimension! Forget your anniversary? Try this and all will be forgiven:

Get her in position Put her in a position where everything is laid out in front of you – lying over a table would work. You need to have easy access to her clitoris, vagina, and anus with your hands and mouth.

Find the AFE Now insert one or two fingers and set sail for the AFE. You're looking for a patch of sensitive skin just above the cervix (yes, that's miles away!) at the innermost point of the vagina. (You can buy long thin vibrators which are curved up at the end which do the job well.)

Find the G-spot Once your fingers (or the vibrator) have gone as far as possible, start stroking what's hopefully the AFE. After a few minutes of stroking, slide your fingers over the front vaginal wall to massage the G-spot (or just the general area if you can't find it) using firm pressure.

Alternate between the two Until she's close to orgasm, alternate between the two techniques, then move in to start licking her clitoris – keeping up the stimulation inside with your fingers. Then insert one well-oiled finger inside her anus for the most explosive orgasm experience she's had in her life. She'll be putty in your hands from now on…

fizzing fellatio

Given the *Kama Sutra* is the most famous sex book in the world, it comes as quite a shock that oral sex barely gets a mention. Vatsyayana may suggest eight different ways to perform fellatio, but the only people supposed to practise it were the "third sex" (gay men) or eunuchs on their masters. Only wanton women or serving maids would stoop so low as to give a man oral pleasure (you hussy, you!) Later, he begrudgingly acknowledged that it was OK between partners of the same social standing if their culture permitted it.

Nevertheless, what little advice is given is good stuff. It concentrates on the art of the tease and adding a bit of spark and variety. Want to add fizz to your fellatio? Here's a sequence based on the original eight ways to perform "mouth congress" – and don't forget to do it in order!

I've renamed the techniques, but the original *Kama Sutra* name is in brackets. Do them in order, and try the pause in-between each to tease him and send his orgasm skyward.

The warm-up (nominal congress) Simply take his penis gently in your mouth and move it about.

Get your teeth into it (biting the sides) Use your hand to hold him still and start nibbling the sides of his penis with your lips. Start with one side, then move down to the other. You're mainly "biting" with your lips, but throw in teensy, gentle nips and see how he responds.

Kiss it better (pressing outside) Did it hurt, diddums? There, there… For this one, you're simply pressing your lips against the head of the penis and kissing it better. A little bit of TLC always goes down well…

Let the teasing begin (pressing inside)   Now put it further into your mouth then "press" it by tightening your lips. Take it out again, then repeat. By the way, for this technique to be effective, he has to relinquish control while you're doing your stuff.

Lip service (kissing)   Hold his penis in your hand, then tuck your bottom lip into the corona, the ridge which separates the head from the shaft. Find his frenulum (the stringy bit) and consistently nudge it with your lower lip. By the way, a lot of these movements are subtle: if he's looking distinctly unimpressed, move swiftly on to the next.

Tongue action (rubbing)   Go for a bit of tongue action – lick his penis all over, then concentrate on tonguing the opening of the urethra (the little hole at the top), pushing your tongue gently into it.

Suck it and see (sucking a mango fruit)   Take him halfway into your mouth, then suck vigorously. I know, I know, sucking is usually considered a schoolgirl error, but after all that teasing, feeling the whole thing enveloped in your warm mouth again will be extraordinary. Sucking hard adds to the contrast between playful licking and serious mouth work. This is why the following is called…

The grand finale (swallowing up)   This isn't quite what it sounds like, because Vatsyayana certainly wouldn't approve of your partner ejaculating in your mouth. By swallowing, he simply meant taking the whole penis into your mouth as if you were trying to swallow it. But by this stage, your partner should be gagging for orgasm, so the chances are you'll wind up swallowing anyway!

By the way, a lot of these movements are subtle: **if he's looking distinctly unimpressed,** move swiftly on to the next.

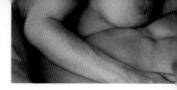

the lowdown on going down

There's fleeting mention of oral sex for him in the *Kama Sutra* – and even less for her! Some say it's because it's biased toward male sexual enjoyment, but I honestly don't believe that. There's so much emphasis on pleasuring women – long, drawn out seductions that take weeks or months to lead to so much as a kiss, and strict instructions on how to read the signs her body is ready for sex before a penis so much as waves at her. For Vatsyayana to avoid instruction on oral sex simply because it's way too much fun for females, doesn't fit. It's far more likely to be for cultural reasons. So why am I bringing it up? Well… hmmm, let's see. One good reason might be because THIS IS HOW MOST WOMEN HAVE ORGASMS! I'm sorry, did I shout that?

He's **taught to read the signs** she's ready before his **penis** so much as **waves** at her.

Even if Vatsyayana didn't wax lyrical about fellatio, he at least threw in a few tricks, which I've dutifully passed on (see pages 58–59). And if the meanie won't deliver on cunnilingus, I will to make things fair! I'm assuming you know the basics (if you don't, my other books *Hot Sex* and *Supersex* both have good guides), so I've just included the juicy bits (so to speak). Read on for what women believe are the crucial steps to getting it right.

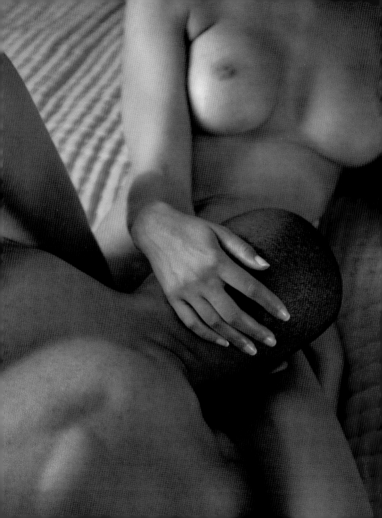

HER TIPS ON GREAT ORAL SEX

Lots of women take up to 20 minutes to orgasm via your tongue, so you are going to need a few ideas to keep you going. Try these techniques in order, or vary them, depending on the reaction you get.

Get comfortable   This could take some time, so get into a position you're comfortable in. The most comfortable position is probably her straddling your face, hanging on to the wall behind, with a pillow or pillows supporting your neck. If she's a bit too shy, pull her over to the edge of the bed and kneel in front of her.

Get some expert advice   Make it abundantly clear you need and want direction from her. While you're getting to know what turns her on, try something for a bit then pull back and ask if she liked it.

Vary the actions   Flicking with a tensed tip of the tongue can feel great, but the most popular technique is to use the whole flat of your tongue and wiggle it or lick, slowly and consistently in between the inner lips and around and over the clitoris.

Read her body language   Lots of women are reluctant to tell you what they want and need, so you need to be alert to her clues. Pay attention to any pressure from her hands if she's holding your head. Pulling you closer means tongue me deeper, pushing you away means you're being too rough. Slow everything down, relax the pressure, and simply lick gently. If she's holding you firmly but seems relaxed, you've got it right.

Change direction   Think about the direction of how you circle her clitoris. It feels quite different clockwise from anti-clockwise. Try mixing it up a little – a few twirls one way, a few twirls the other. As a general rule, the smaller the circle you're making with your tongue, the more intense the stimulation; the larger the circle, the less intense. Start off with large circles, making them smaller as you go along.

Sticking your tongue inside her vagina This can be a huge turn-on, but it's unlikely to make her orgasm. You need to combine it with consistent stimulation of the clitoris. While we are on the subject of penetration, be aware that while some women love you inserting your fingers during oral sex, others find it distracting. How do you find out? You know the answer – ask her!

Stop your tongue getting tired Keep it relaxed rather than tensed, and take little breaks where you move your head rather than your tongue. Or press the flat of it against her clitoris and simply hold it still, letting her move her hips. Make it easier by holding her vaginal lips open and pulling the whole labia up to make her clitoris more visible.

Avoid desensitization Make sure you don't concentrate on exactly the same spot the entire time – unless of course, she wants you to! If she seems to have been enjoying it but isn't now, even though you're doing exactly the same thing, she's probably been over-stimulated to the point of numbness. Reach new spots by drawing a figure of eight on her clitoris, spell her name – or write "Jesus, I wish you'd hurry up because my tongue hurts." Anything to ensure you're hitting a new part of her.

Pace and pressure You may prefer to up the pace and pressure as you approach orgasm, but she may not. A lot of women would rather you continue the same rhythm, which got her close to orgasm in the first place, rather than step it up. Others prefer you to be gentler.

Make noise If you're trying to help tip her over the edge into orgasm, moan to let her know you're as turned on as she is. A brilliant compliment is to say to her: "I almost came when you did, that was such a turn-on."

Throw in some analingus She'll be shy and probably protest the first time around, so take baby steps and work up to a full session. Start by using your tongue tip to play with her clitoris then move to her anus, teasing her clitoris with your fingers at the same time.

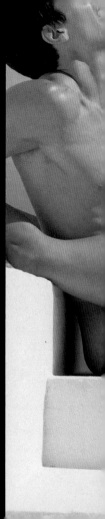

erotic

exotic

exhilarating

exhibitionist

expert

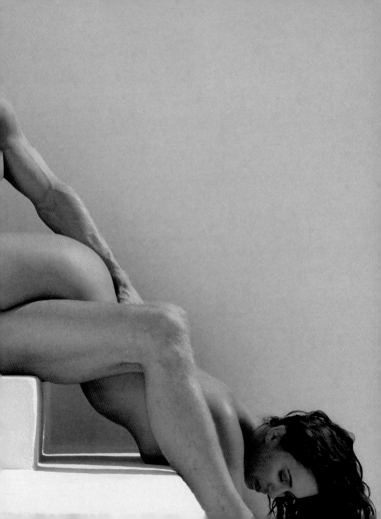

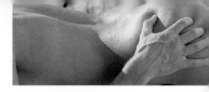

what's your sexual fit?

The way a couple fits together both physically and sexually is taken very seriously by Vatsyayana: compatibility is a central theme of the *Kama Sutra*. To ensure everyone finds their matching sexual bookend, he kindly divides us into three classes dictated by the length of your penis or the size of your vagina. He also helps you predict what's hidden below by how a person looks. And it ain't pretty. There's no faffing about, protecting the delicate male ego or a woman who's self-conscious after giving birth by putting things tactfully or observing any form of political correctness. Vatsyayana cuts straight to the chase.

Well-endowed men get to be proud, mane-tossing, studly "stallions"; guys who weren't first in line when God handed out willy genes are called "hares" – mousy, jittery, fast (and everyone knows that while "a stallion" is on every young girl's wish list, hares never are). And men get it easy. He also describes what you look like so you can find each other. Women with vaginas on the, err… larger side are clumsy, grey, wrinkled old "elephants", while their small sister is a big-eyed, long-limbed, ultra-feminine "doe".

In his defence, Vatsyayana doesn't deliberately set out to upset – or compliment – us. He's simply trying to ensure there's true, pure sexual compatibility. Morbidly curious to know which category you fit into? Read on. The really good news for all of you: it's all a load of bull. Don't take it personally, I just couldn't resist including it for a laugh!

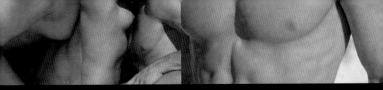

FOR HIM

Hare Around six fingers or approximately 13cm (5in) long. There's no way of putting this delicately, guys: if this is you, you're the smallest. You've got small feet and teensy buttocks, hands, and ears. Your voice is gentle, you've got a round face, and you're always smiling.

Bull Around eight fingers long or approximately 18cm (7in). You're Mr Average. You've also got a thick neck, impressive bearing, red palms, you have an assured air, clear skin, and a nice round tummy.

Stallion About 12 fingers long or approx 25cm (10in). Alright you smug bastard, you knew you'd win. You've also got elongated ears, head, and lips. A thin body, thick hair, long fingers, and heavy thighs. You're a "fast" person and have beautiful nails.

FOR HER

Doe/deer You have a small vagina. You've got beautiful hair, a thin body, narrow face, golden skin, a low voice, and abundant hair.

Mare You have an average vagina. You have wide, strong nostrils and are slightly knock-kneed, with a vagina that is always hot. You've got tender, fat, sweaty arms, regular limbs, a small belly (well that's good), and sexual secretions that smell of meat (not so good). Not surprisingly, given you smell like cooked cow, you're often bad tempered and irritable.

Elephant You have a large vagina. You're tall with a strong body, long teeth, reddish skin, and an unpredictable vagina – sometimes cold and sometimes hot. You talk a lot and your vaginal secretions smell like (wait for it) elephant sweat. There! And you thought the news would be all bad!

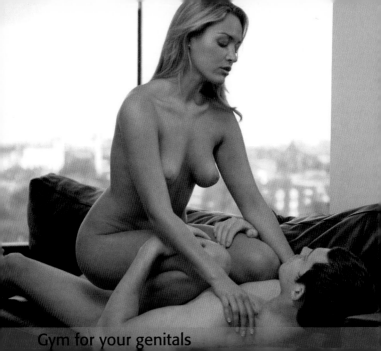

Gym for your genitals

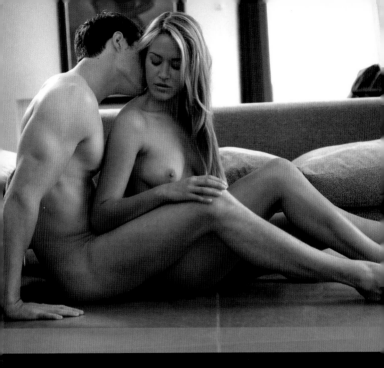

LOVING LEAN

This position can be the prelude to a sex session, or a romantic finale. He sits and she settles between his legs, facing away from him. She then lies back and relaxes against him. He supports his weight on his hands and draws his thighs up to both support and encase her. Bless. We often tend to think of tenderness and passion as mutually exclusive, but they aren't. If you take just one thing from *Kama Sutra*, it's that lesson.

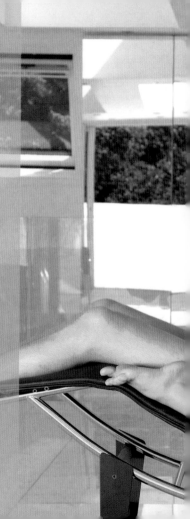

TOP KAMA SUTRA POSITION

tongs

You can both boost your bliss levels with an old favourite! Vatsyayana was all for women being in control.

How to do it

Nothing too fancy about this one – it's your basic woman-on-top! He lies back and relaxes, she sits on top of him, knees bent. It's called the "tongs" because instead of lifting herself up and down, she's squeezing his penis repeatedly with her vaginal muscles, moving it in and out rather like someone using a pair of tongs! If you fancy a change, grind in circular movements. This feels great for him and stimulates her clitoris.

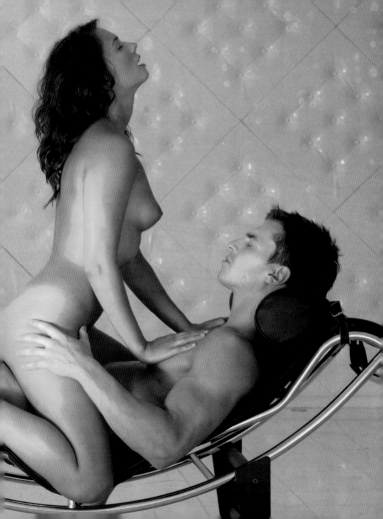

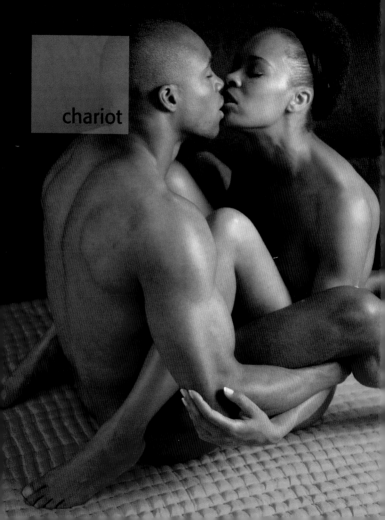

chariot

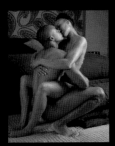

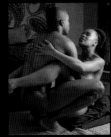

^^STEP ONE

Get yourselves to a cushy surface; it'll pay off later. He squats, she lowers herself on to his penis to sit in his lap and snog him sexily.

<<STEP TWO

Staying inside her, he tips her backwards. She supports herself by holding on to his back, he also holds on tight. This position dramatically alters the angle of her vagina.

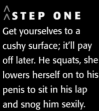

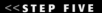

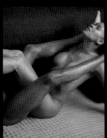

<<STEP THREE

Dropping on to the soft surface, both extend your legs, placing them near or on each other's shoulders, supporting your own weight on your elbows.

<<STEP FIVE

… And that's the moment when it makes perfect sense to shift into the relaxing final position. Erotically knitted together, it's time to see-saw your way to orgasm.

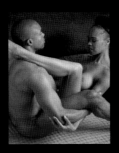

<<STEP FOUR

Sitting up to move closer, he widens his thighs as you both link arms underneath his knees. His feet are on the floor to steady you as you both rock.

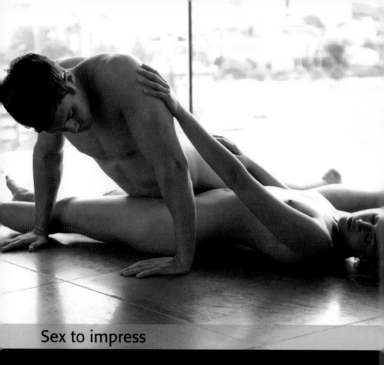

Sex to impress

THE SWIVEL

Want to really impress her? Start in the basic missionary
position but just as she's starting to think "How predictable",
you pull back, look deep into her eyes… and prepare to move.
Lift one leg, then the other so both your legs are on one side of
her, keeping your penis inside. Move your hands and feet until
your body lies sideways across hers. Keep moving until you're
facing her toes, carefully lifting your leg over her head.

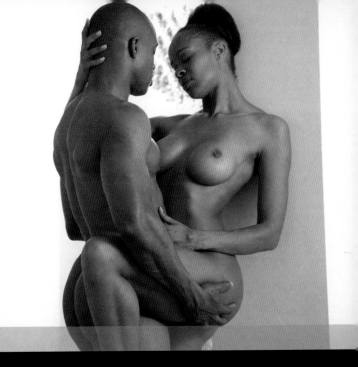

THE VINE

This one is a bit of a carnal challenge, but for fast, urgent,
spontaneous sex you can't beat it. She leans against a wall,
lifting one leg to help him penetrate and he stands between
her thighs, holding her raised leg under her bottom and upper
thigh. She leans into the wall for stability and to allow him to
thrust away with abandon. The higher she lifts her leg on his
thigh, the deeper the penetration.

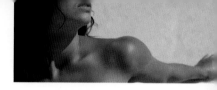

cosmic coming

This technique is what every spiritual sex student really enrols for: the legendary whole-body orgasm (WBO). There's a lot of hype surrounding this one: some pooh-pooh the whole concept, others claim it's the most powerful experience of their lives. The difference between a WBO and your average garden variety is you'll feel it throughout your body, not just centred in your genital area. Picture wave-like pulsations of energy surging from head to toe and you'll get some idea of what it feels like. Bring it on? Yes! The basic idea is to get to the "almost" stage a couple of times before you orgasm. Try these exercises to get an idea of what you're in for.

FOR HIM

Get control Masturbate until you're highly aroused, then stop and contract your PC muscle – the one that moves your penis up and down.

Calm it down Concentrate on keeping your heart rate as low as possible, breathing slowly and calmly.

Build up the pressure Continue masturbating and repeat the whole process a couple of times. Imagine you're drawing the sexual energy up your spine, away from your genitals. Keep your breathing calm and even.

Contract that PC muscle As you feel yourself hit 8–9 on a scale of 1–10 for orgasm (10 being lift off), stop, contract your PC again and visualize the energy shooting to your brain, through your whole body.

Explode! If you feel an orgasm still have an erection, you've done it! It takes practice, though. Often years of it!

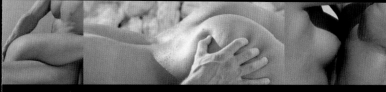

FOR HER

Relax Get your head in the right place. Make sure you're focused and ready to let your mind go and your body take over.

Masturbate Arouse yourself by masturbating, using erotica or fantasizing, or get him to start stimulating you. Consciously relax and clear your mind of anything but the pleasure and excitement you're feeling.

Focus on your clitoris Use your fingers, a vibrator (or his fingers or tongue!) Let yourself move steadily toward orgasm, but when you get too close stop all stimulation for just a moment. Then continue.

Have your first orgasm Tip over into orgasm land, this one courtesy of the clitoris. As the waves begin (and immediately afterward), squeeze your anus tight, pump those pelvic floor (PC) muscles, and imagine sending all that orgasmic energy up your spine. Keep breathing.

Open your channels Touch your tongue to the roof of your mouth, half an inch behind your front teeth. Doing this allows the sexual energy to flow freely throughout your body for a WBO.

Build up to another orgasm To try for another orgasm, this time in the vagina, focus on bringing that energy back to your genitals again. Start stimulating the clitoris again within 30 seconds of the first orgasm. Use the teasing technique you used before.

Want multiples? Now start stimulating the clitoris and vagina simultaneously. Use a vibrator, your fingers or his to penetrate, working particularly on the front vaginal wall. As this is happening, start squeezing your pelvic floor muscles rhythmically to focus energy in your vagina. Keep going and – bonus! – you should have a vaginal orgasm.

erotic

exotic

exhilarating

exhibitionist

—

expert

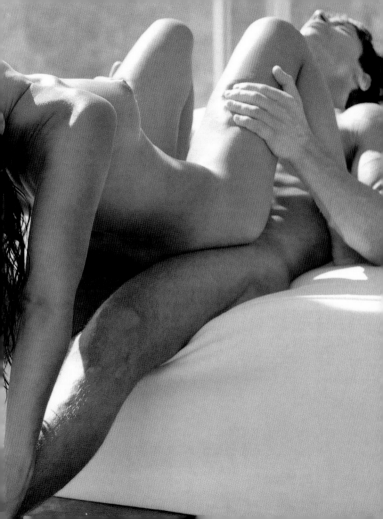

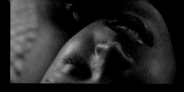

take the plunge

Forget what the history books tell you, in the *Kama Sutra* sexual equality existed 2,000 years ago. Vatsyayana portrays females as sensual, sexual beings who are able to, and should, initiate and take control during sex.

A prime purpose of the *Kama Sutra* is to teach men to be sensitive, skilful lovers who understand the sexual needs of women. Vatsyayana realized the female sexual system was different to a man's – and he recognized that women are more instinctive about sex than men, needing less formal instruction because of our strongly developed sense of intuition.

The ultimate aim is to keep it inside for 100 heartbeats. Since both your hearts will be **thudding away like buggery,** this isn't as long as it sounds.

Most importantly, the *Kama Sutra* teaches women not to be ashamed of sex or desire. For instance, her hopping on top to take control – both of penetration and her orgasm – is perfectly OK. Thought you'd get to lie back while he did all the work? Hah! You've obviously never read any of my books before. Here are some expert thrusting techniques for you to try, too. He will be very impressed, and you get to control the orgasms.

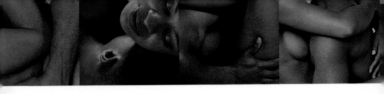

THRUSTING FOR HER

The next time you're on top (yes, it does mean effort, but trust me, it pays off!) try fast or slow rocking, moving your hips in slow circles, and raising or lowering onto him at different speeds. If you mix up your thrusting style, the average bout of intercourse is going to be one hell of a lot more interesting. It not only makes you look sexually savvy and erotically experienced, it ups your chance of having an orgasm through penetration only, and feels damn good for him, too. Here's a few ideas:

The (pair of) tongs Clench your PC muscles and hold his penis inside you as tight as you possibly can. Grip, squeeze, and internally stroke it by "milking" (think the rhythmic ritual of milking a cow – squeeze and release, squeeze and release).

The top You turn around on the man's body like a wheel so that your back is towards him. Yes, this isn't one to be tackled half-heartedly. Think lots of practice, giggles, and training and you're about one-fifth there.

The bee Crouch in a sitting position over him and revolve your vagina around his penis while he arches his back to make it easier. "Easier" said with tongue-in-cheek: this is an advanced technique (but it's not so far out there you shouldn't attempt it!).

The swing Sway in wide circles over him, using your whole body to make a figure of eight. Again, ambitious but doable – give it a go!

Melting together When you feel tired of being the boy, lie down on top of him and rest without breaking coital contact. That's the whole point of spiritual sex – there's no reason to rush. To get things going again, move gently to restimulate his penis (and your bits, too).

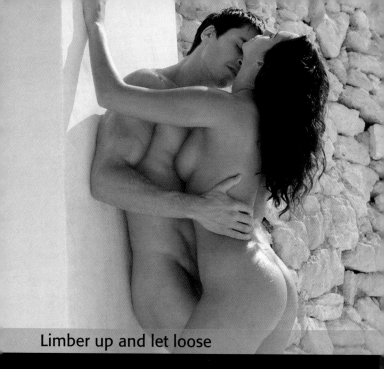

Limber up and let loose

STAND AND DELIVER

This position looks deceptively easy, until you stop to think about the angle at which he's penetrating her. Some men find this one uncomfortable because his penis is bent awkwardly, and unless she keeps her bottom well and truly tilted back and upward, he tends to pop out rather frequently. So why should you try it? Because if you get it right, it's a brilliant position for one of those spur-of-the-moment shags!

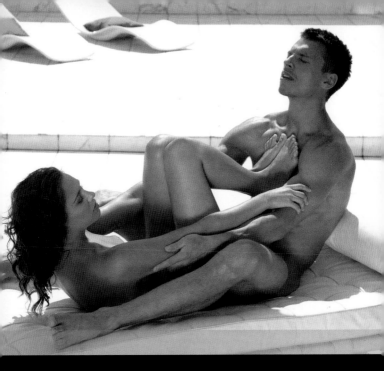

CHEST PRESS

Start with both of you sitting up straight. She puts her feet on his chest and leans back to allow him to penetrate, then both of you hold on to each other's arms and lean backwards. If you were to do this one strictly by the book, he'd also put his feet on her chest. (If you manage this, contact the *Guinness Book of Records* immediately!) Not surprisingly, the only "thrusting" option you have in this position is to rock back and forth

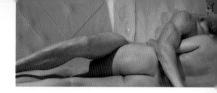

get your teeth into it

In *Kama Sutra* time, leaving scratches, bites, or other marks of passion in a place where everyone could see them was very much the done thing – a passionate stamp of sexual ownership. These days, turning up to work with a whopping great love-bite on your neck isn't recommended as a great career move. But in Vatsyayana's time, marking was not only a way of ensuring nobody stole what was yours (the whole "If you love someone set them free" thing wasn't huge back then), it was designed to give your lover something to remember you by while you were gone, evoking not just hot flushes of lust, but love.

Biting, particularly for women, was encouraged as a way to show their partner they really were enjoying themselves, rather than faking it. Though, as Vatsyayana points out, it was usually women "of a passionate nature" who did it and it was more likely to happen on certain occasions: the first time a couple have sex, before they're about to be parted, when they're reunited, during "make up" sex – and if a woman is drunk!

Whichever way you look at it, scratching and biting is animalistic – which means lusty types will love it and the more timid will find it horribly intimidating. I'd say it's safe to assume most people won't really want to advertise what they did the night before by being marked in a place that's on view. But if you're talking doing it in a private place where only your partner can see it, well, that can be absurdly erotic.

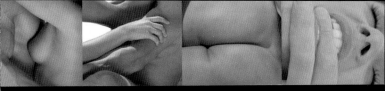

LEAVING YOUR MARK

A few (rather obvious) rules if you want to try this out on your partner: make sure they're happy to be marked, agree on where is off limits, and only do it when they're *über* turned on. A bite out of the blue will get you slapped rather than snogged. Here are some marks and bites to try:

MARKS

Sounding Simply dragging your nails across your lover's skin to make the hairs stand up. This should be done on the breasts and thighs.

Half moon Push your nails into their skin making crescent-shaped marks. Use this technique on their neck, breast, or chest.

A line Draw your nails down the back.

Tiger claw A scratch resembling a tiger claw which curves over the surface of her breast.

BITES

The hidden bite Your classic love bite left in a hidden place, such as on the neck, breast, or chest.

The point A nip taken with just two teeth.

Coral and jewel Biting with your teeth and using pressure from your lips on their cheek or bottom cheek. (I'd be going for the second option if I were you.) Lips are perceived as coral and the teeth as jewels.

The line of jewels Biting using all your teeth.

Biting of the boar Literally taking a piece out of your partner. Only to be done by and to people of great passion (ie randy little buggers).

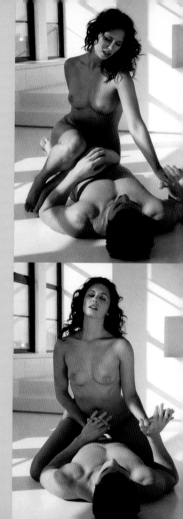

07
TOP KAMA SUTRA POSITION

spinning top

This involves her sitting on his penis, then swivelling herself all the way around on it like a spinning top. Yes, it is totally bonkers!

How to do it

Even Vatsyayana strongly urges you to practise this lots (like, no kidding!), but if you break it down into stages it can work in a wobbly type of way! She starts by assuming the usual her-on-top position then (very slowly and carefully) lifts one leg over his body so both her legs are on one side. The next move is to turn her body so she's now facing away from him. Just be careful for God's sake!

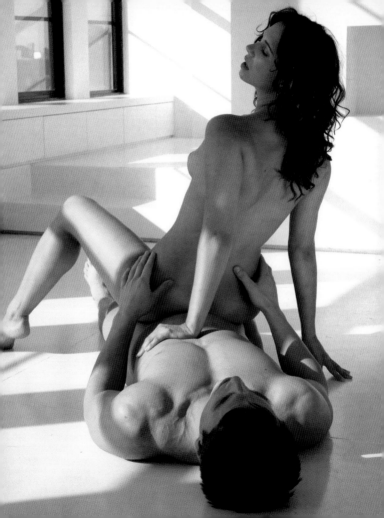

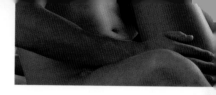

the really naughty bits

Want to know how to please five women at once, or the etiquette for threesomes? The *Kama Sutra* doesn't seem to worry about social taboos as we do today. Vatsyayana doesn't just acknowledge wanting to covet your neighbour's wife, he gives detailed instructions. Cheating is OK, he had no qualms about pre-marital sex, and he cheerfully instructs men on how to sneak into a harem. Here are some highlights:

THREESOMES AND GROUP SEX

Non-judgemental and ridiculously liberal, he obligingly describes the correct etiquette for threesomes and group sex – down to the minutest detail. There's a particularly raunchy passage where Vatsyayana talks about how women in country villages hide young men in their apartments with "highly sensual women sometimes hiding several". Greedy girlies!

The men satiate the women's desires either one by one or as a group: "One holds her seated on his knees, while another takes her mouth and embraces her. One bites and scratches her, while the other penetrates her sex or licks her vulva. She is scratched, bitten, and beaten separately by one after the other, or by all together, after which they fornicate with her successively. One of the practices that satisfies a woman and calms the excitation of her hole of pleasure, the opening for the passage of liquids, or vulva, consists of one of them servicing her sex with his mouth." Well, I don't know about you but it made me wiggle a little in my seat!

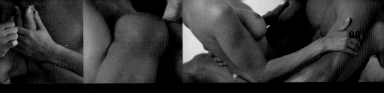

He's not sexist either: "In the same way, this can be done by the women of the King's harem when they accidentally get hold of a man." Just how you "accidentally" get hold of a man, sadly, isn't explained.

Samghataka rata is the term for having a threesome: a man making love with two women "who like each other and have the same taste" (whether this refers to clothes, men, or furniture isn't specified). "The two women lie on the same bed and the boy makes use of them both. While he is mounting one, the other, excited, kisses him and after pleasuring one he brings the other to orgasm." Threesomes also worked the other way around with two men and one woman.

The prize for "The Least Likely Sex Scenario" to happen now in real life goes to the '"Congress of a Herd of Cows" – one man satisfying five women at one time. Princes and rich merchants might well have been able to enjoy this, but for your average man today, it will probably remain a fantasy. But just in case you do find yourself surrounded by five naked, willing women, here's his advice… You lie in front of three women, giving one of them oral sex and spreading your arms to put your fingers deep inside the two other women flanking her. At the same time, you're penetrating a fourth woman who is lying underneath you with her head at the opposite end to yours. A fifth girl sits on top of the fourth girl's face, receiving cunnilingus. A cinch! (A warning though for any couples reading this and feeling curious: group sex may be best left as a fantasy. It's quite rare for both partners to love it, and very few can handle the jealousy.)

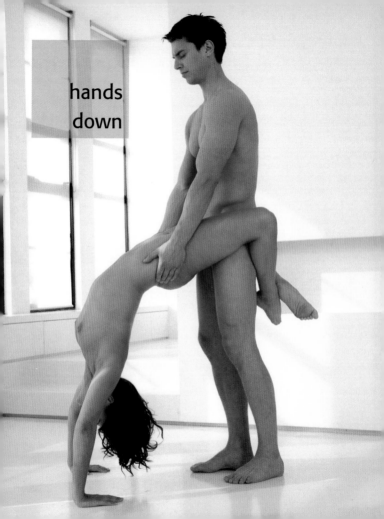

hands
down

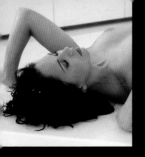

STEP ONE

Start with her flat on the floor, her bottom raised and feet in line with her hips. She then brings her hands up by her ears, turning them so her fingertips point downwards.

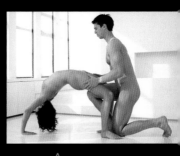

^STEP TWO

She arches her back, lifting her hips in the air. He supports her as she arches, kneeling on one leg.

<<STEP FOUR

He completely straightens up and she crosses her feet behind his back. It's up to him to move her back and forth. Good luck!

<<STEP THREE

He stands up s-l-o-w-l-y, still holding on tight to her, moving his hands to support her lower back. He takes mos of the strain, not her

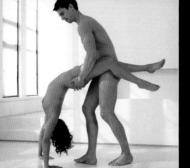

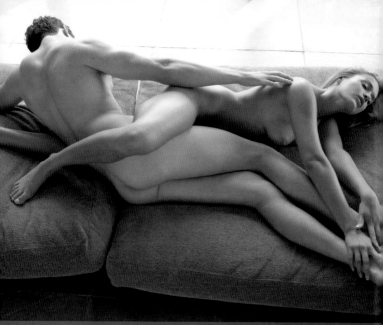

Flash positions for frisky lovers

TOP-TO-TOE

This looks damn impressive but the truth is, if you've had side-by-side sex, you've probably done a similar version without even realizing it. The only difference is, instead of facing the same way, you're lying in opposite directions (heads pointed towards each other's feet). Thing is, most women move down the bed to make penetration easier and this simply exaggerates that natural movement. It's easy, it's fun, it's familiar. Go for it!

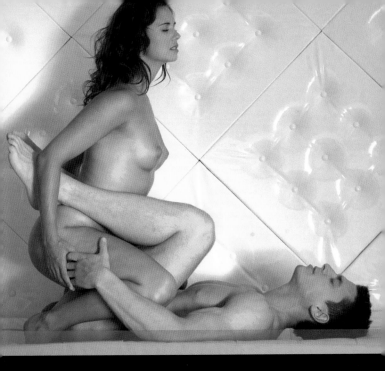

THE HORSE RIDE

This position is inspired by horse riding, he lies on his back and draws his knees up, parting his thighs. She wiggles between them, using her hand to help insert his penis, then leans forward, using her knees to move up and down on his penis, "riding" him like he's a horse. Putting firm cushions under his shoulders can make this easier. If her legs start to get tired, he can sit up while she sits back so you're sitting face to face.

index

acknowledgements

This is my seventh book about sex, and my 11th book in total, and I'm extremely happy to say I have had the pleasure of working with pretty much the same people for each one. I've thanked you all profusely in the past, but just in case you haven't got the message of how much I treasure you all…

To my family, Shirley, Terry, Patrick, Maureen, Nigel, Diana, Deborah, Doug, Charlie, and Maddy. They say families aren't perfect but by God, you come close!

To my agent and best friend, Vicki McIvor. Humblest thanks, as always, for being such a support in my life in all ways possible. I am so lucky to have you!

To all my closest, dearest friends, Sandra Aldridge, Peggy Bunker, Rachel Corcoran, Claire Faragher, Catherine Jarvie, and Fenella Thomas. Thanks for being so patient with me, even though we all know I'm a workaholic, and for making me laugh even when stress levels were at their highest.

To the couples who road-tested positions. I know you don't want to be named, but surely it's obvious who you are from the various unexplained injuries?

To my editor, Dawn Bates, for not only doing a superb job (as usual), but for laughing at all my jokes (even those you rather swiftly edited out).

To Peter Jones at DK, who's been there with me from the start and never once failed to be outstandingly supportive and ridiculously patient. Thanks for always humouring me.

To my book designers, Nigel Wright and Bev Speight at XAB, for turning my words into such a visual treat.

To Stephanie Jackson at DK, for being such an enthusiastic fan of my work and inspiration for me to come up with even more funky, fresh new titles.

And to all at Dorling Kindersley, world-wide, enormous thanks for everything. In the UK office, John Roberts, Deborah Wright, Serena Stent, Hermoine Ireland, Liz Statham, Catherine Bell, Adèle Hayward, Helen Spencer, and Katherine Raj. In the US office, Gary June, Therese Burke, Tom Korman, and Rachel Kempster, and in Canada, Chris Houston and Loraine Taylor.

DK would like to thank Laurence Errington for indexing, Clare Hubbard for proof-reading, and Katherine Raj for design assistance.

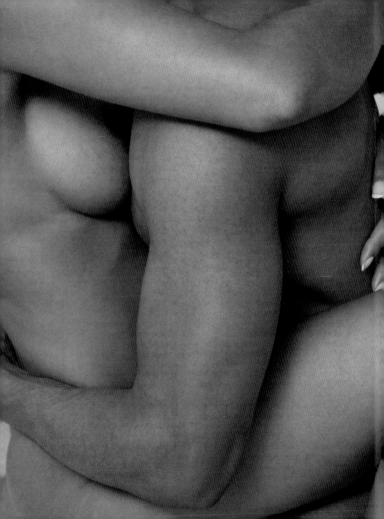